I'M VERY Ferris

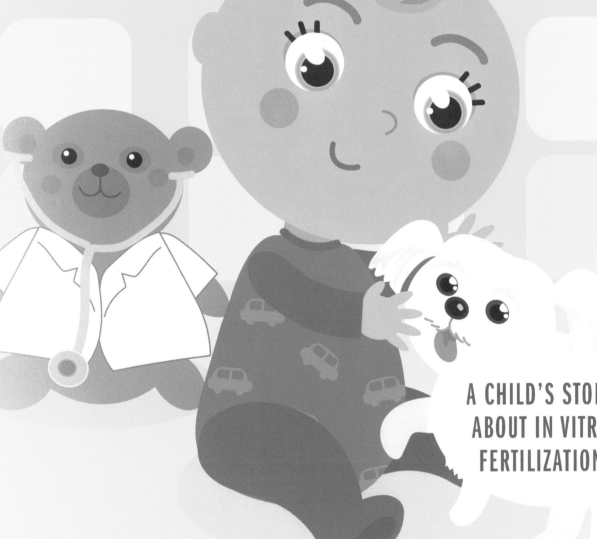

A CHILD'S STORY
ABOUT IN VITRO
FERTILIZATION

TESS KOSSOW

D0851137

I'm Very Ferris
A Child's Story About In Vitro Fertilization
All Rights Reserved.
Copyright © 2019 Tess Kossow
v2.0

The opinions expressed in this manuscript are solely the opinions of the author and do not represent the opinions or thoughts of the publisher. The author has represented and warranted full ownership and/or legal right to publish all the materials in this book.

This book may not be reproduced, transmitted, or stored in whole or in part by any means, including graphic, electronic, or mechanical without the express written consent of the publisher except in the case of brief quotations embodied in critical articles and reviews.

Outskirts Press, Inc.
http://www.outskirtspress.com

Paperback ISBN: 978-1-9772-0067-9
Hardback ISBN: 978-1-9772-0466-0

Library of Congress Control Number: 2018911653

Illustrated by: Carla Castagno.
Illustrations © 2019 Outskirts Press, Inc. All rights reserved - used with permission.

Outskirts Press and the "OP" logo are trademarks belonging to Outskirts Press, Inc.

PRINTED IN THE UNITED STATES OF AMERICA

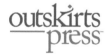

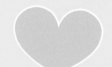

This Book
Belongs to:

Jackson

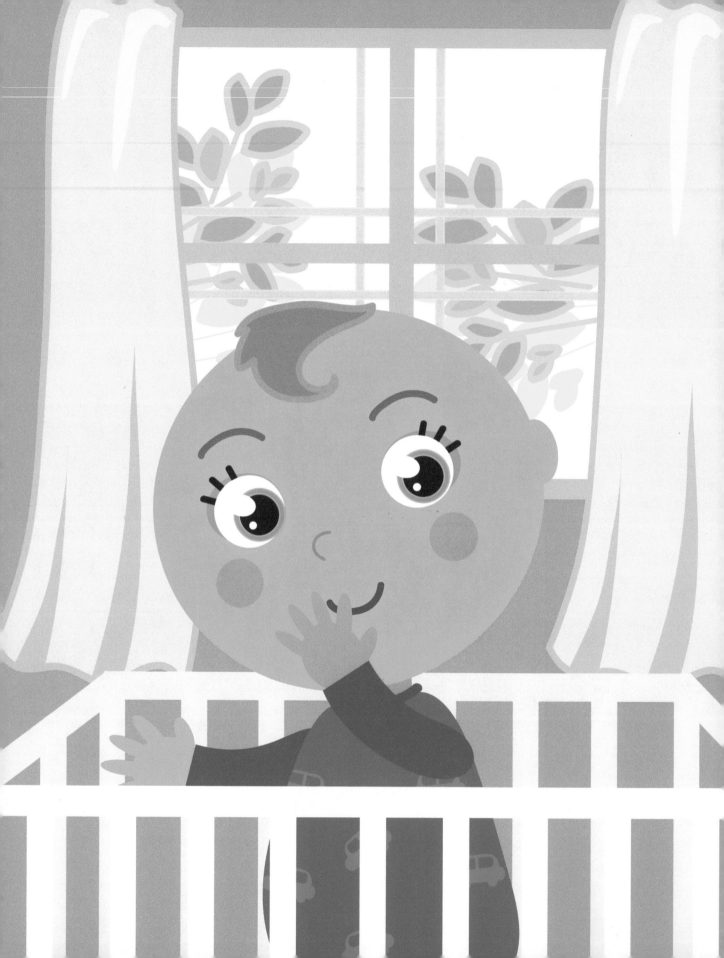

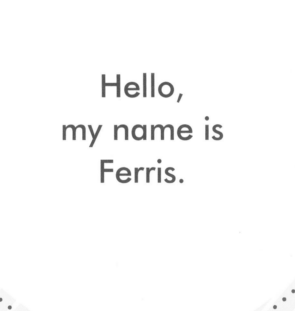

Hello,
my name is
Ferris.

I'm like other babies,
but with a special story
about my birth.

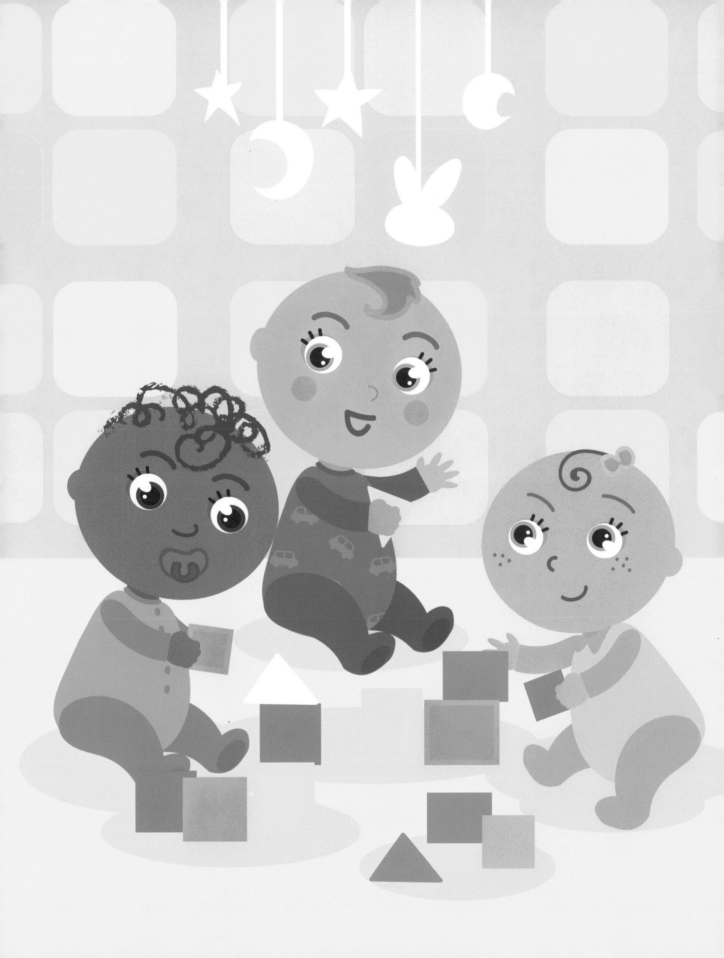

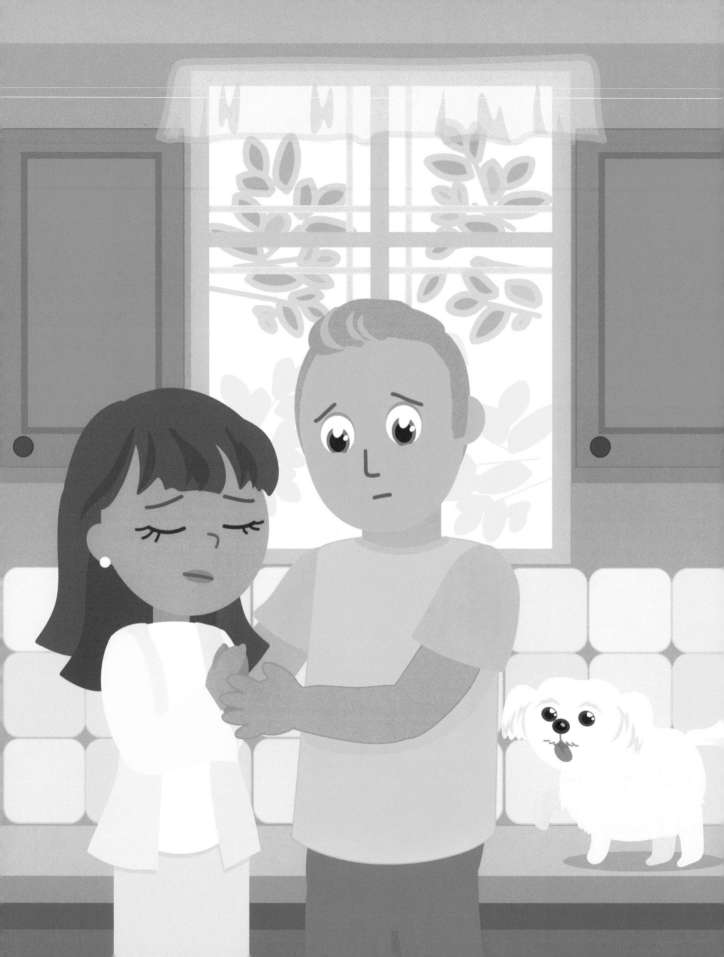

Mama and Dad
prayed, wished, and
tried to create me,

but needed help
from an infertility doctor
on Earth.

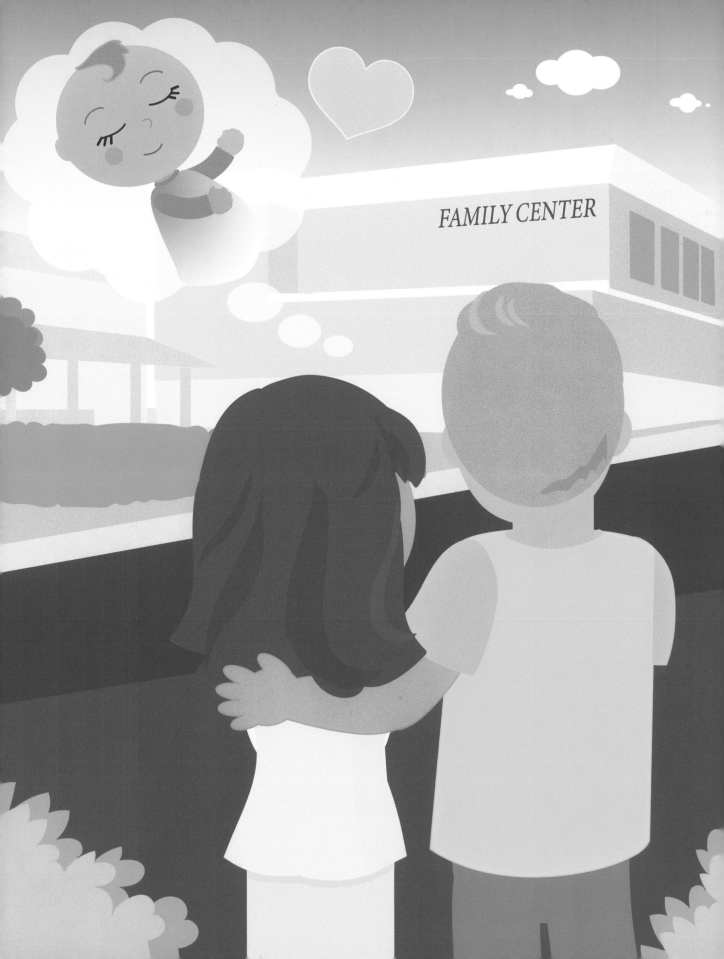

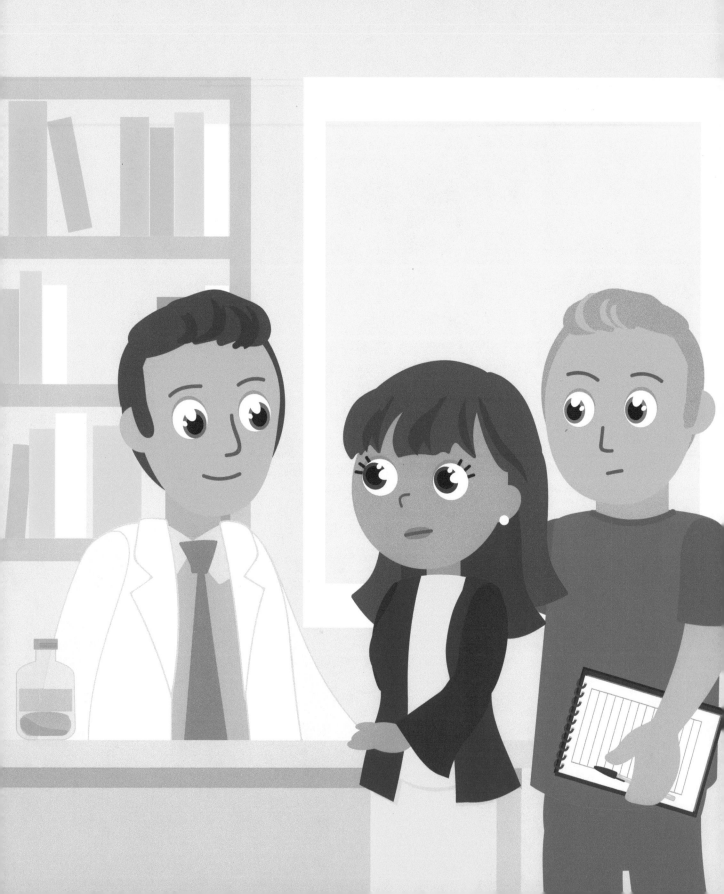

A doctor who joined
Mama's egg
and Dad's genes

to create, with
the power of medicine
and success, me!

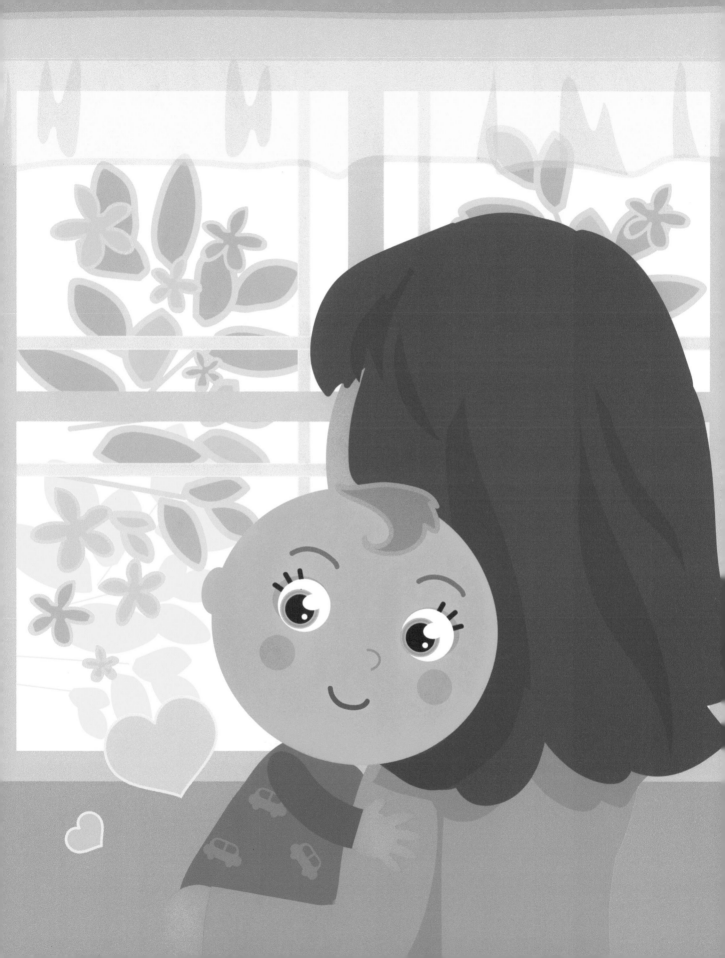

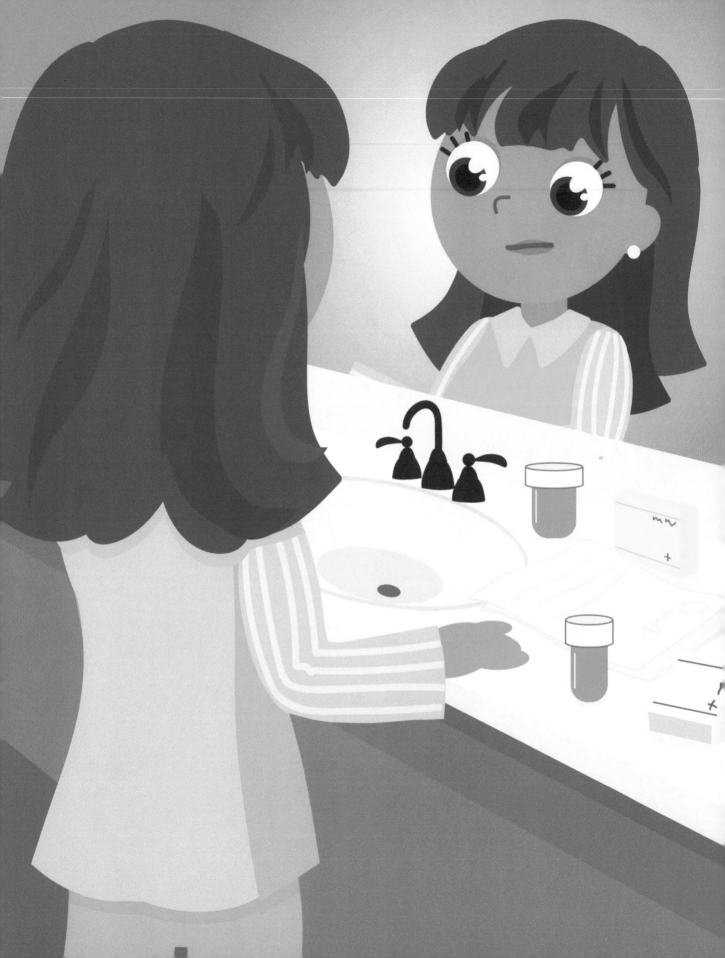

It wasn't easy,
and I did not happen
overnight.

Mama had surgeries,
and lots of shots,
to make her body right.

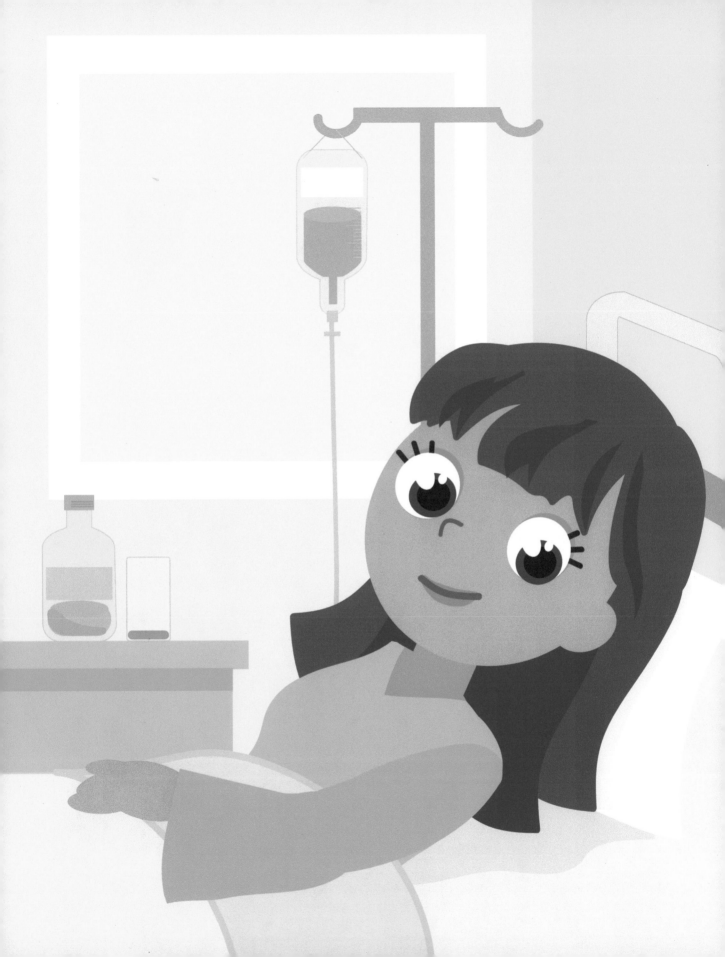

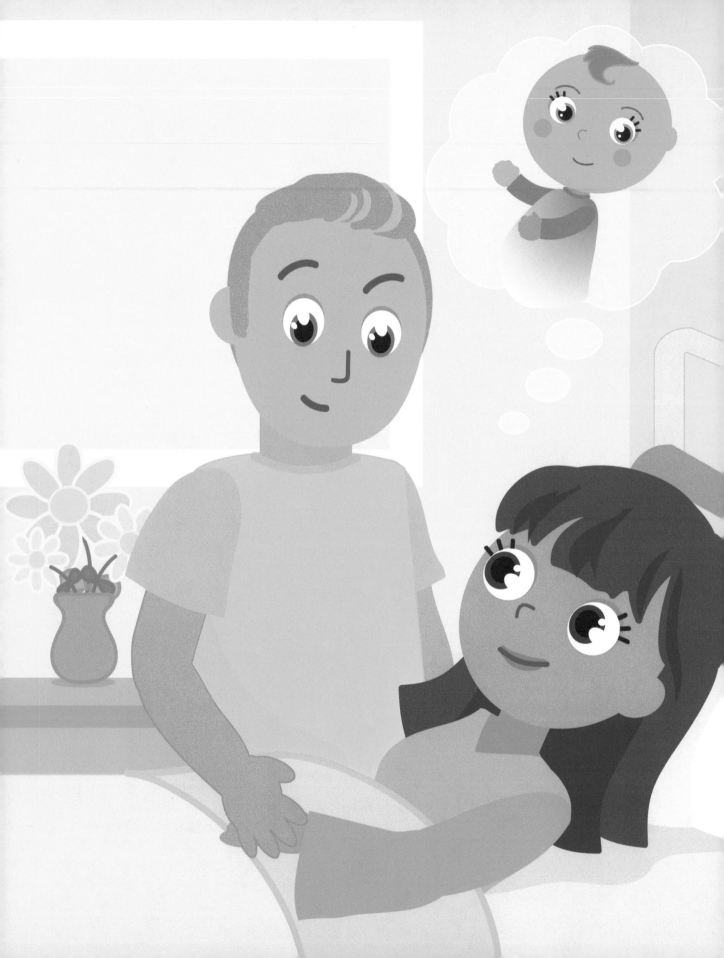

With Dad
by Mama's side,
and all genetic
tests a go,

the infertility doctor
transferred me,
a healthy embryo.

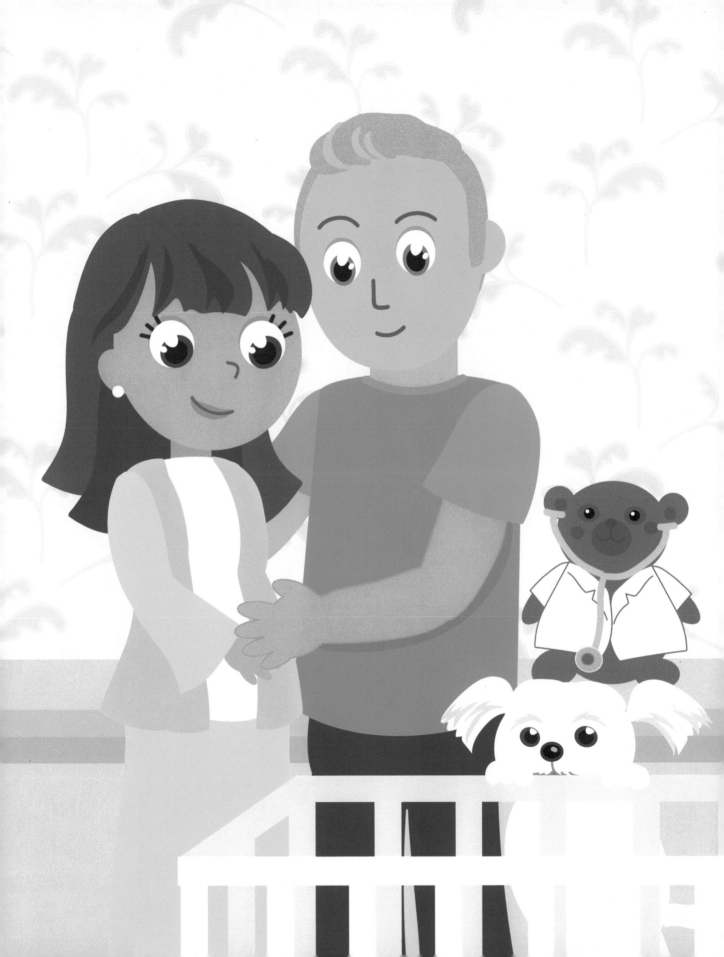

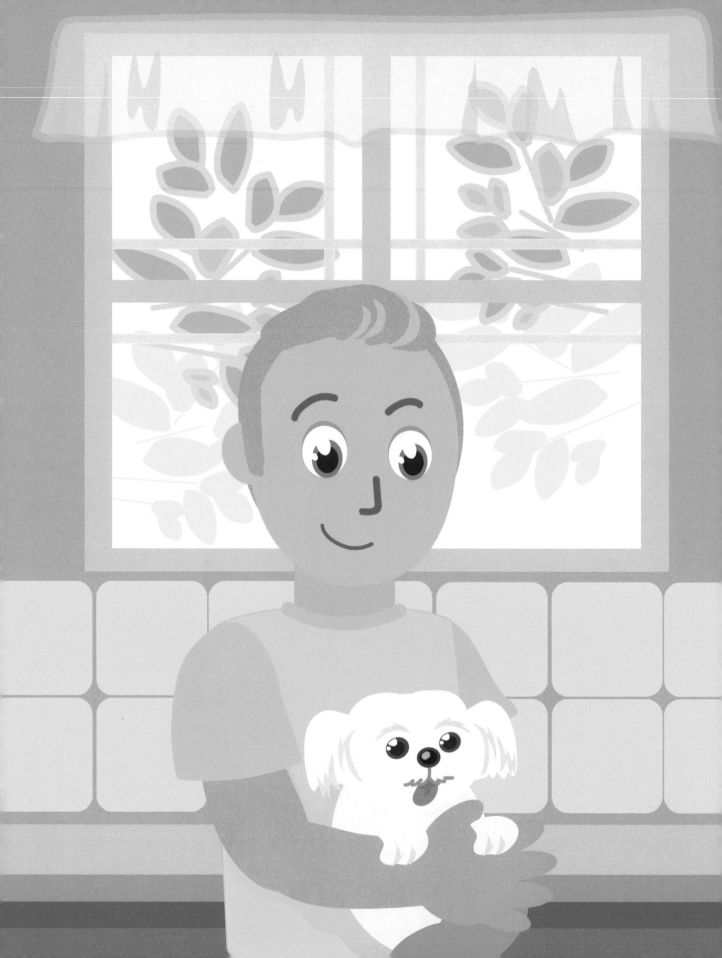

Mama and Dad
took a risk with faith

that with positive thoughts, they would have their own baby someday.

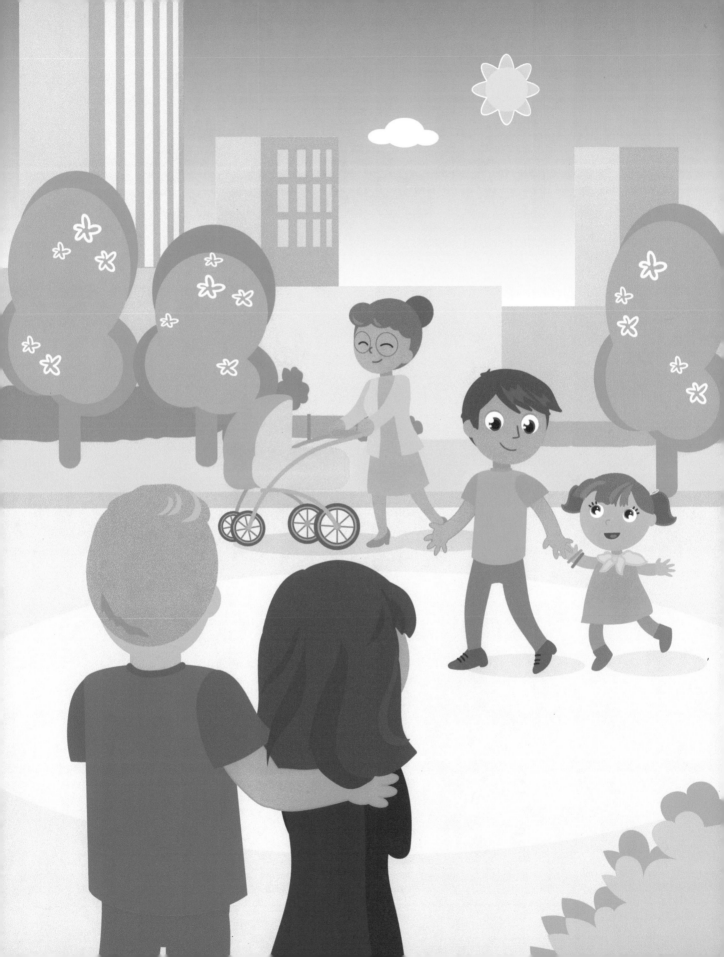

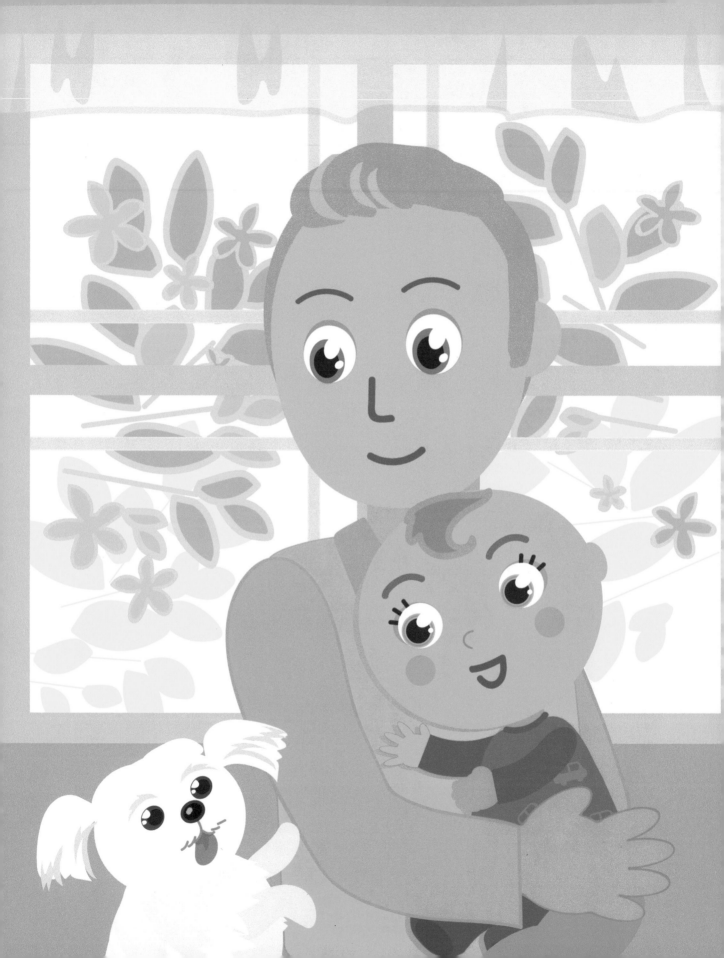

And at 39 weeks,
they welcomed a boy
with endless kisses
and hugs.

My parents named
me Ferris and are so
thankful to have me
to love.

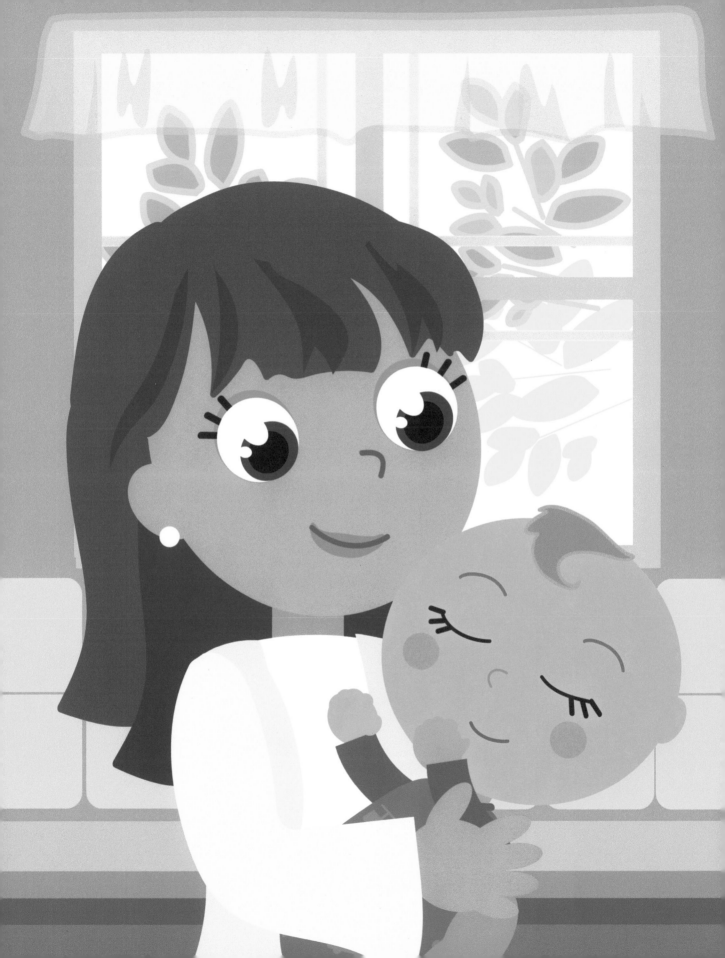

CPSIA information can be obtained
at www.ICGtesting.com
Printed in the USA
LVHW072224221119
638245LV00004B/38/P